WEIGHT LOSS T

MONTH:

DATE	WEIGHT	GAIN+	LOSS+	NOTES

WEIGHT LOSS TRACKER

MONTH: YEAR:

DATE	WEIGHT	GAIN+	LOSS+	NOTES

WEIGHT LOSS TRACKER

MONTH: YEAR:

DATE	WEIGHT	GAIN+	LOSS+	NOTES

WEIGHT LOSS TRACKER

MONTH: YEAR:

DATE	WEIGHT	GAIN+	LOSS+	NOTES

WEIGHT LOSS TRACKER

MONTH: YEAR:

DATE	WEIGHT	GAIN+	LOSS+	NOTES

WEIGHT LOSS TRACKER

MONTH: YEAR:

DATE	WEIGHT	GAIN+	LOSS+	NOTES

WEIGHT LOSS TRACKER

MONTH: YEAR:

DATE	WEIGHT	GAIN+	LOSS+	NOTES

WEIGHT LOSS TRACKER

MONTH: YEAR:

DATE	WEIGHT	GAIN+	LOSS+	NOTES

WEIGHT LOSS TRACKER

MONTH: YEAR:

DATE	WEIGHT	GAIN+	LOSS+	NOTES

WEIGHT LOSS TRACKER

MONTH: YEAR:

DATE	WEIGHT	GAIN+	LOSS+	NOTES

WEIGHT LOSS TRACKER

MONTH: YEAR:

DATE	WEIGHT	GAIN+	LOSS+	NOTES

WEIGHT LOSS TRACKER

MONTH: YEAR:

DATE	WEIGHT	GAIN+	LOSS+	NOTES

WEIGHT LOSS TRACKER

MONTH: YEAR:

DATE	WEIGHT	GAIN+	LOSS+	NOTES

WEIGHT LOSS TRACKER

MONTH: YEAR:

DATE	WEIGHT	GAIN+	LOSS+	NOTES

WEIGHT LOSS TRACKER

MONTH: YEAR:

DATE	WEIGHT	GAIN+	LOSS+	NOTES

WEIGHT LOSS TRACKER

MONTH: YEAR:

DATE	WEIGHT	GAIN+	LOSS+	NOTES

WEIGHT LOSS TRACKER

MONTH: YEAR:

DATE	WEIGHT	GAIN+	LOSS+	NOTES

WEIGHT LOSS TRACKER

MONTH: YEAR:

DATE	WEIGHT	GAIN+	LOSS+	NOTES

WEIGHT LOSS TRACKER

MONTH: YEAR:

DATE	WEIGHT	GAIN+	LOSS+	NOTES

WEIGHT LOSS TRACKER

MONTH: YEAR:

DATE	WEIGHT	GAIN+	LOSS+	NOTES

WEIGHT LOSS TRACKER

MONTH: YEAR:

DATE	WEIGHT	GAIN+	LOSS+	NOTES

WEIGHT LOSS TRACKER

MONTH: YEAR:

DATE	WEIGHT	GAIN+	LOSS+	NOTES

WEIGHT LOSS TRACKER

MONTH: YEAR:

DATE	WEIGHT	GAIN+	LOSS+	NOTES

WEIGHT LOSS TRACKER

MONTH: YEAR:

DATE	WEIGHT	GAIN+	LOSS+	NOTES

WEIGHT LOSS TRACKER

MONTH: YEAR:

DATE	WEIGHT	GAIN+	LOSS+	NOTES

WEIGHT LOSS TRACKER

MONTH: YEAR:

DATE	WEIGHT	GAIN+	LOSS+	NOTES

WEIGHT LOSS TRACKER

MONTH: YEAR:

DATE	WEIGHT	GAIN+	LOSS+	NOTES

WEIGHT LOSS TRACKER

MONTH: YEAR:

DATE	WEIGHT	GAIN+	LOSS+	NOTES

WEIGHT LOSS TRACKER

MONTH: YEAR:

DATE	WEIGHT	GAIN+	LOSS+	NOTES

WEIGHT LOSS TRACKER

MONTH: YEAR:

DATE	WEIGHT	GAIN+	LOSS+	NOTES

WEIGHT LOSS TRACKER

MONTH: YEAR:

DATE	WEIGHT	GAIN+	LOSS+	NOTES

WEIGHT LOSS TRACKER

MONTH: YEAR:

DATE	WEIGHT	GAIN+	LOSS+	NOTES

WEIGHT LOSS TRACKER

MONTH: YEAR:

DATE	WEIGHT	GAIN+	LOSS+	NOTES

WEIGHT LOSS TRACKER

MONTH: YEAR:

DATE	WEIGHT	GAIN+	LOSS+	NOTES

WEIGHT LOSS TRACKER

MONTH: YEAR:

DATE	WEIGHT	GAIN+	LOSS+	NOTES

WEIGHT LOSS TRACKER

MONTH: YEAR:

DATE	WEIGHT	GAIN+	LOSS+	NOTES

WEIGHT LOSS TRACKER

MONTH: YEAR:

DATE	WEIGHT	GAIN+	LOSS+	NOTES

WEIGHT LOSS TRACKER

MONTH: YEAR:

DATE	WEIGHT	GAIN+	LOSS+	NOTES

WEIGHT LOSS TRACKER

MONTH: YEAR:

DATE	WEIGHT	GAIN+	LOSS+	NOTES

WEIGHT LOSS TRACKER

MONTH: YEAR:

DATE	WEIGHT	GAIN+	LOSS+	NOTES

WEIGHT LOSS TRACKER

MONTH: YEAR:

DATE	WEIGHT	GAIN+	LOSS+	NOTES

WEIGHT LOSS TRACKER

MONTH: YEAR:

DATE	WEIGHT	GAIN+	LOSS+	NOTES

WEIGHT LOSS TRACKER

MONTH: YEAR:

DATE	WEIGHT	GAIN+	LOSS+	NOTES

WEIGHT LOSS TRACKER

MONTH: YEAR:

DATE	WEIGHT	GAIN+	LOSS+	NOTES

WEIGHT LOSS TRACKER

MONTH: YEAR:

DATE	WEIGHT	GAIN+	LOSS+	NOTES

WEIGHT LOSS TRACKER

MONTH: YEAR:

DATE	WEIGHT	GAIN+	LOSS+	NOTES

WEIGHT LOSS TRACKER

MONTH: YEAR:

DATE	WEIGHT	GAIN+	LOSS+	NOTES

WEIGHT LOSS TRACKER

MONTH: YEAR:

DATE	WEIGHT	GAIN+	LOSS+	NOTES

WEIGHT LOSS TRACKER

MONTH: YEAR:

DATE	WEIGHT	GAIN+	LOSS+	NOTES

WEIGHT LOSS TRACKER

MONTH: YEAR:

DATE	WEIGHT	GAIN+	LOSS+	NOTES

WEIGHT LOSS TRACKER

MONTH: YEAR:

DATE	WEIGHT	GAIN+	LOSS+	NOTES

WEIGHT LOSS TRACKER

MONTH: YEAR:

DATE	WEIGHT	GAIN+	LOSS+	NOTES

WEIGHT LOSS TRACKER

MONTH: YEAR:

DATE	WEIGHT	GAIN+	LOSS+	NOTES

WEIGHT LOSS TRACKER

MONTH: YEAR:

DATE	WEIGHT	GAIN+	LOSS+	NOTES

WEIGHT LOSS TRACKER

MONTH: YEAR:

DATE	WEIGHT	GAIN+	LOSS+	NOTES

WEIGHT LOSS TRACKER

MONTH: YEAR:

DATE	WEIGHT	GAIN+	LOSS+	NOTES

WEIGHT LOSS TRACKER

MONTH: YEAR:

DATE	WEIGHT	GAIN+	LOSS+	NOTES

WEIGHT LOSS TRACKER

MONTH: YEAR:

DATE	WEIGHT	GAIN+	LOSS+	NOTES

WEIGHT LOSS TRACKER

MONTH: YEAR:

DATE	WEIGHT	GAIN+	LOSS+	NOTES

WEIGHT LOSS TRACKER

MONTH: YEAR:

DATE	WEIGHT	GAIN+	LOSS+	NOTES

WEIGHT LOSS TRACKER

MONTH: YEAR:

DATE	WEIGHT	GAIN+	LOSS+	NOTES

WEIGHT LOSS TRACKER

MONTH: YEAR:

DATE	WEIGHT	GAIN+	LOSS+	NOTES

WEIGHT LOSS TRACKER

MONTH: YEAR:

DATE	WEIGHT	GAIN+	LOSS+	NOTES

WEIGHT LOSS TRACKER

MONTH: YEAR:

DATE	WEIGHT	GAIN+	LOSS+	NOTES

WEIGHT LOSS TRACKER

MONTH: YEAR:

DATE	WEIGHT	GAIN+	LOSS+	NOTES

WEIGHT LOSS TRACKER

MONTH: YEAR:

DATE	WEIGHT	GAIN+	LOSS+	NOTES

WEIGHT LOSS TRACKER

MONTH: YEAR:

DATE	WEIGHT	GAIN+	LOSS+	NOTES

WEIGHT LOSS TRACKER

MONTH: YEAR:

DATE	WEIGHT	GAIN+	LOSS+	NOTES

WEIGHT LOSS TRACKER

MONTH: YEAR:

DATE	WEIGHT	GAIN+	LOSS+	NOTES

WEIGHT LOSS TRACKER

MONTH: YEAR:

DATE	WEIGHT	GAIN+	LOSS+	NOTES

WEIGHT LOSS TRACKER

MONTH: YEAR:

DATE	WEIGHT	GAIN+	LOSS+	NOTES

WEIGHT LOSS TRACKER

MONTH: YEAR:

DATE	WEIGHT	GAIN+	LOSS+	NOTES

WEIGHT LOSS TRACKER

MONTH: YEAR:

DATE	WEIGHT	GAIN+	LOSS+	NOTES

WEIGHT LOSS TRACKER

MONTH: YEAR:

DATE	WEIGHT	GAIN+	LOSS+	NOTES

WEIGHT LOSS TRACKER

MONTH: YEAR:

DATE	WEIGHT	GAIN+	LOSS+	NOTES

WEIGHT LOSS TRACKER

MONTH: YEAR:

DATE	WEIGHT	GAIN+	LOSS+	NOTES

WEIGHT LOSS TRACKER

MONTH: YEAR:

DATE	WEIGHT	GAIN+	LOSS+	NOTES

WEIGHT LOSS TRACKER

MONTH: YEAR:

DATE	WEIGHT	GAIN+	LOSS+	NOTES

WEIGHT LOSS TRACKER

MONTH: YEAR:

DATE	WEIGHT	GAIN+	LOSS+	NOTES

WEIGHT LOSS TRACKER

MONTH: YEAR:

DATE	WEIGHT	GAIN+	LOSS+	NOTES

WEIGHT LOSS TRACKER

MONTH: YEAR:

DATE	WEIGHT	GAIN+	LOSS+	NOTES

WEIGHT LOSS TRACKER

MONTH: YEAR:

DATE	WEIGHT	GAIN+	LOSS+	NOTES

WEIGHT LOSS TRACKER

MONTH: YEAR:

DATE	WEIGHT	GAIN+	LOSS+	NOTES

WEIGHT LOSS TRACKER

MONTH: YEAR:

DATE	WEIGHT	GAIN+	LOSS+	NOTES

WEIGHT LOSS TRACKER

MONTH: YEAR:

DATE	WEIGHT	GAIN+	LOSS+	NOTES

WEIGHT LOSS TRACKER

MONTH: YEAR:

DATE	WEIGHT	GAIN+	LOSS+	NOTES

WEIGHT LOSS TRACKER

MONTH: YEAR:

DATE	WEIGHT	GAIN+	LOSS+	NOTES

WEIGHT LOSS TRACKER

MONTH: YEAR:

DATE	WEIGHT	GAIN+	LOSS+	NOTES

WEIGHT LOSS TRACKER

MONTH: YEAR:

DATE	WEIGHT	GAIN+	LOSS+	NOTES

WEIGHT LOSS TRACKER

MONTH: YEAR:

DATE	WEIGHT	GAIN+	LOSS+	NOTES

WEIGHT LOSS TRACKER

MONTH: YEAR:

DATE	WEIGHT	GAIN+	LOSS+	NOTES

WEIGHT LOSS TRACKER

MONTH: YEAR:

DATE	WEIGHT	GAIN+	LOSS+	NOTES

WEIGHT LOSS TRACKER

MONTH: YEAR:

DATE	WEIGHT	GAIN+	LOSS+	NOTES

WEIGHT LOSS TRACKER

MONTH: YEAR:

DATE	WEIGHT	GAIN+	LOSS+	NOTES

WEIGHT LOSS TRACKER

MONTH: YEAR:

DATE	WEIGHT	GAIN+	LOSS+	NOTES

WEIGHT LOSS TRACKER

MONTH: YEAR:

DATE	WEIGHT	GAIN+	LOSS+	NOTES

WEIGHT LOSS TRACKER

MONTH: YEAR:

DATE	WEIGHT	GAIN+	LOSS+	NOTES

WEIGHT LOSS TRACKER

MONTH: YEAR:

DATE	WEIGHT	GAIN+	LOSS+	NOTES

WEIGHT LOSS TRACKER

MONTH: YEAR:

DATE	WEIGHT	GAIN+	LOSS+	NOTES

WEIGHT LOSS TRACKER

MONTH: YEAR:

DATE	WEIGHT	GAIN+	LOSS+	NOTES

Printed in Great Britain
by Amazon

36026270R00056